PREDIABETES COOKBOOK FOR BEGINNERS

SAMANTHA WOOLERY

Contents

INTRODUCTION.. 9

  My Story 9

OVERVIEW OF PREDIABETES............................ 14

  Understanding Prediabetes 14

  Making Positive Lifestyle Changes.................. 14

PREDIABETES BASICS 16

  Risk Factors For Prediabetes: 16

  Symptoms And Diagnosis:.............................. 17

  Nutrition Essentials for Prediabetes............... 18

  Carbohydrates And Blood Sugar Control........ 21

  Glycemic Index And Glycemic Load:............... 22

  Fiber And Blood Sugar Control: 23

  Importance Of Fiber:..................................... 25

  Healthy Fats And Protein: 26

  Portion Control And Mindful Eating: 27

MEAL PLANNING AND PREPPING...................... 29

  Creating A Meal Plan:.................................... 29

  Grocery Shopping Tips: 30

  Meal Prepping Strategies: 31

Batch Cooking And Freezing:...................... 32

Smart Snacking Options: 33

BREAKFAST AND BRUNCH RECIPES 34

Energizing Breakfast Bowls 34

Tropical Acai Bowl:................................. 34

Berry Quinoa Breakfast Bowl: 36

Green Smoothie Bowl: 37

Overnight Chia Pudding Bowl:.................... 38

Greek Yogurt Breakfast Bowl: 39

Peanut Butter Banana Oatmeal Bowl:........ 40

Mexican Breakfast Bowl:........................... 41

Mediterranean Egg Breakfast Bowl:........... 42

Flavorful Omelets And Frittatas 44

Spinach and Feta Omelet: 44

Mushroom and Swiss Cheese Frittata: 46

Mediterranean Vegetable Omelet: 47

Bacon and Cheddar Frittata: 49

Tomato and Basil Omelet:........................ 51

NUTRITIOUS SMOOTHIES AND SHAKES:............. 53

Green Detox Smoothie:............................. 53

Berry Blast Smoothie: 55

Tropical Mango Smoothie:........................... 56

Peanut Butter Banana Protein Shake: 57

Chocolate Avocado Protein Smoothie:.......... 58

LUNCH AND DINNER RECIPES 60

Nourishing Soups And Salads Urishing Soups: 60

Lentil Soup: 60

Chicken Noodle Soup: 62

Tomato Basil Soup: 64

Butternut Squash Soup: 65

Minestrone Soup:............................ 67

Turkey Avocado Wrap:...................... 69

Caprese Panini: 70

Greek Chicken Pita: 72

Vegetarian Quinoa Salad Wrap: 73

Wholesome Grain And Vegetable Bowls:....... 76

Quinoa and Roasted Vegetable Bowl: 76

Brown Rice and Teriyaki Tofu Bowl: 78

Quinoa and Chickpea Power Bowl:............. 79

Farro and Grilled Vegetable Bowl:............. 81

Barley and Roasted Beet Bowl: 82

Lemon Garlic Roasted Chicken: 83

DELICIOUS VEGETARIAN AND VEGAN OPTIONS. 85

Lentil Curry: 85

Vegetable Stir-Fry: 87

Chickpea And Vegetable Curry: 89

Zucchini Noodles With Pesto: 91

Vegan Black Bean Tacos: 93

SNACKS AND SIDES 96

Healthy Snack Ideas 96

Greek Yogurt Parfait: 96

Vegetable Sticks with Hummus: 98

Hard-Boiled Egg and Whole Grain Crackers:99

Apple Slices with Almond Butter: 100

Avocado Toast: 100

Trail Mix: 101

Cottage Cheese with Berries: 102

Cucumber and Tomato Salad: 103

Edamame: 104

Rice Cakes with Nut Butter: 104

LIFESTYLE TIPS FOR MANAGING PREDIABETES 106

Incorporating Physical Activity: 106

Stress Management Techniques: 107

Importance Of Sleep And Rest: 108

Building A Supportive Network: 110

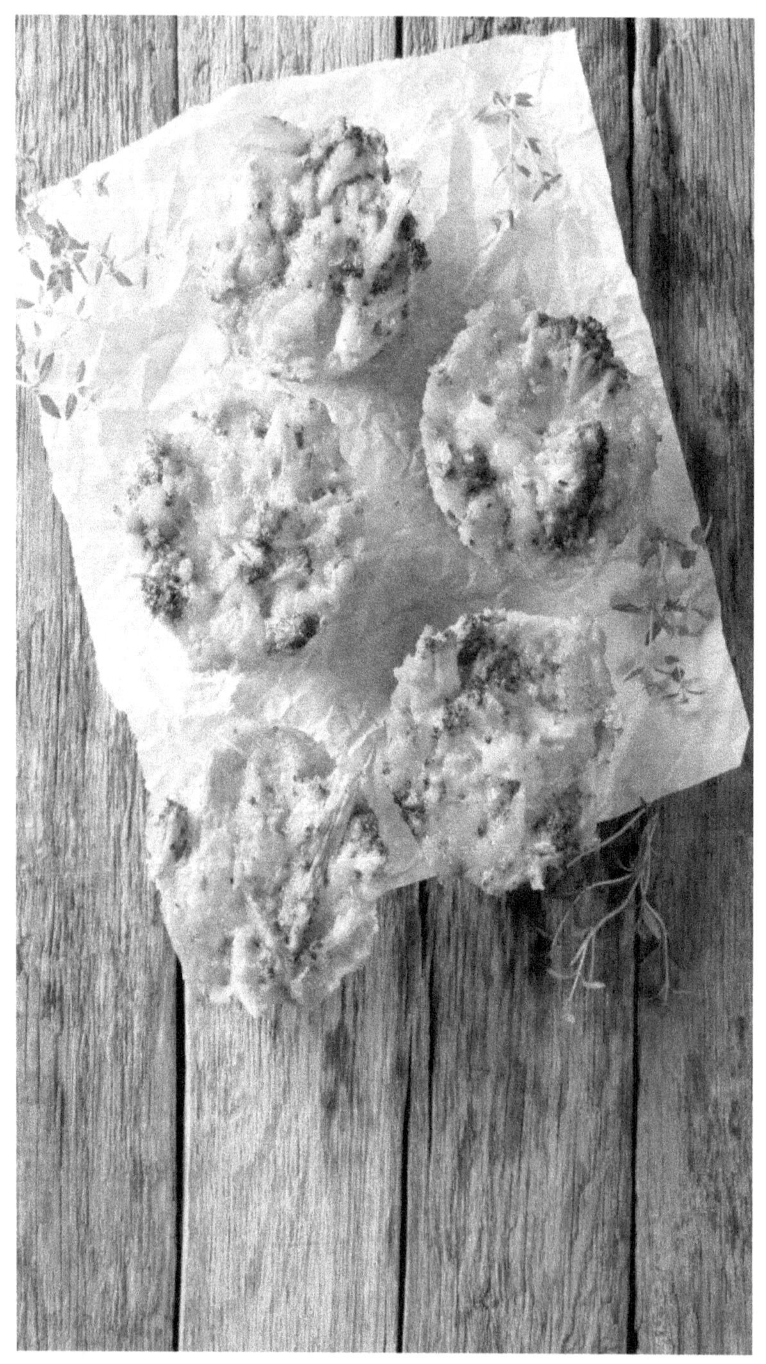

INTRODUCTION

My Story

Once upon a time in the bustling city of New York, lived Emily, a vibrant young woman who had recently been diagnosed with prediabetes. Filled with determination, Emily embarked on a journey to take control of her health and prevent the progression of her condition. She knew that making significant changes to her diet and lifestyle was crucial, but she felt overwhelmed and unsure of where to begin.

One day, while browsing through a local bookstore, Emily stumbled upon a beautifully designed cookbook titled "The Prediabetes Cookbook for Beginners." Intrigued, she picked it up and began to explore its pages. The table of contents caught her attention, promising a comprehensive guide to managing prediabetes through delicious and nutritious recipes.

Excited by the prospect of having a resource tailored specifically to her needs, Emily purchased the cookbook and eagerly dove into its contents. The first chapter, "Prediabetes Basics," answered all of Emily's questions. She learned about the definition and risk factors associated with prediabetes, enabling her to better comprehend her own situation. Armed with this knowledge, Emily felt empowered and motivated to take charge of her health.

Moving on to the next section, "Nutrition Essentials for Prediabetes," Emily discovered a wealth of information on building a balanced plate, understanding carbohydrates, and incorporating healthy fats and proteins into her diet. The cookbook emphasized the importance of portion control and mindful eating, teaching her to make mindful choices that would help stabilize her blood sugar levels.

With newfound knowledge, Emily tackled the chapter on meal planning and prepping. It provided her with practical tips for creating a personalized meal plan, navigating the grocery store, and efficiently prepping meals for the week. Armed with a list of smart snacking options, she felt confident in her ability to maintain a healthy diet throughout her busy schedule.

But it was the recipes that truly transformed Emily's culinary journey. The cookbook offered a wide range of breakfast, lunch, and dinner ideas that were not only delicious but also tailored to prediabetes management. Emily experimented with energizing breakfast bowls, flavorful omelets, and satisfying grain bowls. She marveled at the creativity of the recipes, which transformed mundane ingredients into culinary delights.

Snacks and sides became a delightful part of Emily's day, with healthy options that satisfied her cravings without compromising her health. She relished guilt-free dips and spreads, relishing in the flavors of nutritious vegetable and fruit sides. Even desserts and treats were not off-limits. Emily delighted in sugar-free and low-sugar delights, savoring indulgent occasional delights while still staying within her dietary limits.

As Emily incorporated the recipes into her daily routine, she began noticing positive changes in her health. Her energy levels increased, and she experienced fewer spikes in her blood sugar levels. She felt a sense of control over her condition and embraced a healthier lifestyle.

Not only did the cookbook provide Emily with nourishing recipes, but it also offered lifestyle tips for managing prediabetes. She learned the importance of incorporating physical activity, managing stress, and prioritizing quality sleep. The cookbook became her trusted companion, guiding her towards a better and healthier life.

As Emily reflected on her journey, she realized that the Prediabetes Cookbook for Beginners had been her guiding light. It had provided her with the knowledge, inspiration, and practical tools she needed to make positive changes in her diet and lifestyle. It had empowered her to take control of her health and prevent the progression of prediabetes.

Filled with gratitude, Emily decided to share her story with others who were also facing the challenges of prediabetes. She became an advocate for healthy living, hosting cooking workshops and sharing her favorite recipes from the cookbook. Through her efforts, she inspired countless individuals to embrace a healthier lifestyle and provided them with the invaluable resource that had transformed her life—the Prediabetes Cookbook for Beginners.

In the end, Emily's journey served as a testament to the power of knowledge, support, and delicious recipes in managing prediabetes. With the right tools and a strong determination, anyone could turn their health around and enjoy a fulfilling life. The Prediabetes Cookbook for Beginners had become more than just a book to Emily—it had become a symbol of hope, empowerment, and a recipe for health.

Welcome to the Prediabetes Cookbook for Beginners, a comprehensive guide designed to empower you on your journey towards managing prediabetes and embracing a healthier lifestyle. Whether you've recently been diagnosed with prediabetes or simply want to take proactive steps to prevent its onset, this cookbook is here to provide you with valuable knowledge, practical tips, and delicious recipes that will support your well-being.

OVERVIEW OF PREDIABETES

Understanding Prediabetes

Prediabetes is a condition characterized by higher than normal blood sugar levels, but not high enough to be diagnosed as type 2 diabetes. It is considered an intermediate stage between normal blood sugar levels and diabetes. Prediabetes is a significant warning sign that indicates an increased risk of developing type 2 diabetes in the future.

When a person has prediabetes, their body either does not produce enough insulin or becomes resistant to the insulin it does produce. Insulin is a hormone produced by the pancreas that helps regulate the amount of sugar (glucose) in the bloodstream and facilitates its transfer into cells for energy production.

Making Positive Lifestyle Changes

Healthy Eating Habits:

Adopting a nutritious and balanced eating plan is crucial for managing prediabetes. Focus on consuming whole foods, such as fruits, vegetables, whole grains, lean proteins, and healthy fats. Incorporate fiber-rich foods, as they help regulate blood sugar levels and promote a feeling of fullness. Limit the intake of refined carbohydrates, sugary foods, and beverages, as they can cause rapid spikes in blood sugar levels. Portion control is also essential, as maintaining a healthy weight plays a significant role in prediabetes management.

Regular Physical Activity:

Engaging in regular physical activity is a powerful tool in managing prediabetes. Exercise helps improve insulin sensitivity, allowing your body to use glucose more effectively. Aim for at least 150 minutes of moderate-intensity aerobic activity per week, such as brisk walking, cycling, or swimming. Additionally, incorporate strength training exercises at least twice a week to build muscle mass and further enhance insulin sensitivity. Find activities you enjoy and make them a regular part of your routine.

PREDIABETES BASICS

Risk Factors For Prediabetes:

Prediabetes can affect individuals of any age, gender, or background. Understanding the risk factors associated with prediabetes can help identify those who may be at higher risk and take preventive measures. Some common risk factors include:

Excess Weight: Being overweight or obese is a significant risk factor for prediabetes. The excess body fat, especially around the abdomen, can contribute to insulin resistance and impair glucose regulation.

Sedentary Lifestyle: Leading a sedentary lifestyle with little to no physical activity increases the risk of developing prediabetes. Lack of regular exercise can contribute to weight gain, reduced insulin sensitivity, and impaired glucose metabolism.

Family History: Having a close family member with type 2 diabetes, such as a parent or sibling, increases the risk of prediabetes. Genetics play a role in the development of the condition, although lifestyle factors also contribute.

Age: The risk of prediabetes tends to increase with age, especially after the age of 45. This may be due to a natural decline in insulin sensitivity and changes in body composition that occur as we get older.

Gestational Diabetes: Women who have had gestational diabetes during pregnancy are at higher risk of developing prediabetes later in life. It also increases the risk of type 2 diabetes in the future.

High Blood Pressure: Having high blood pressure (hypertension) is associated with an increased risk of prediabetes. Both conditions often coexist and share common underlying risk factors.

Symptoms And Diagnosis:

Prediabetes often does not cause noticeable symptoms, which is why it often goes undiagnosed. However, some individuals may experience mild symptoms such as increased thirst, frequent urination, fatigue, and blurred vision. These symptoms are not specific to prediabetes and can be attributed to other factors as well.

Prediabetes is typically diagnosed through blood tests that measure blood sugar levels. The most common tests used for diagnosis are:

Fasting Plasma Glucose (FPG) Test: This test measures blood glucose levels after an overnight fast. A fasting blood sugar level between 100 and 125 mg/dL is indicative of prediabetes.

Oral Glucose Tolerance Test (OGTT): During this test, blood sugar levels are measured after fasting and again two hours after consuming a glucose-rich drink. A two-hour blood sugar level between 140 and 199 mg/dL indicates prediabetes.

Nutrition Essentials for Prediabetes

Building a Balanced Plate

A balanced plate is the cornerstone of a healthy and nutritious diet. It involves selecting a variety of foods from different food groups to provide the essential nutrients your body needs to function properly. By building a balanced plate, you can support overall well-being, maintain a healthy weight, and reduce the risk of chronic diseases, including prediabetes and type 2 diabetes. Here are some key principles to consider when building a balanced plate:

Fill Half Your Plate with Colorful Vegetables and Fruits:

Vegetables and fruits are rich in vitamins, minerals, antioxidants, and dietary fiber. They should form the foundation of your balanced plate. Aim to fill at least half of your plate with a variety of colorful and non-starchy vegetables and fruits. These include leafy greens, broccoli, bell peppers, berries, citrus fruits, and more. They provide essential nutrients while being low in calories and high in fiber, which aids digestion, promotes satiety, and helps regulate blood sugar levels.

Incorporate Whole Grains:

Choose whole grains over refined grains to ensure a higher fiber content and a lower glycemic index. Whole grains include options like whole wheat, brown rice, quinoa, oats, and whole grain bread and pasta. They provide important vitamins, minerals, and fiber, which support digestive health and help control blood sugar levels. Aim to make at least half of your grain intake whole grains.

Include Lean Proteins:

Protein is essential for the growth, repair, and maintenance of tissues in the body. Choose lean sources of protein such as skinless poultry, fish, beans, lentils, tofu, and low-fat dairy products. These options provide high-quality protein while being lower in saturated fat and cholesterol. Including protein in your meals helps promote satiety, stabilize blood sugar levels, and support muscle health.

Healthy Fats in Moderation:

Incorporate healthy fats into your balanced plate, but remember to consume them in moderation. Healthy fat sources include avocados, nuts, seeds, olive oil, and fatty fish like salmon and trout. These fats provide essential fatty acids, vitamins, and antioxidants that contribute to heart health and overall well-being. However, they are calorie-dense, so portion control is important.

Carbohydrates And Blood Sugar Control

Types of Carbohydrates:

Carbohydrates can be categorized into two main types: simple carbohydrates and complex carbohydrates.

a. Simple Carbohydrates: Simple carbohydrates are quickly digested and rapidly increase blood sugar levels. These include foods and beverages with added sugars, such as soft drinks, candies, pastries, and desserts. Consuming excessive amounts of simple carbohydrates can lead to blood sugar spikes, which can be detrimental for individuals with prediabetes. It's important to limit or avoid these sources of simple carbohydrates as much as possible.

b. Complex Carbohydrates: Complex carbohydrates are digested more slowly and have a gentler impact on blood sugar levels. They contain more fiber, vitamins, and minerals compared to simple carbohydrates. Complex carbohydrates can be found in whole grains (e.g., whole wheat, oats, quinoa), legumes (e.g., lentils, chickpeas, kidney beans), starchy vegetables (e.g., sweet potatoes, butternut squash), and some fruits. These sources of complex carbohydrates are nutrient-dense and provide a steady release of glucose into the bloodstream, helping to maintain more stable blood sugar levels.

Glycemic Index And Glycemic Load:

The glycemic index (GI) is a scale that ranks carbohydrates based on how quickly they raise blood sugar levels. Foods having a high GI value (70 or above) are swiftly broken down and result in a greater rise in blood sugar. Low GI foods (those with a GI of 55 or below) are digested more gradually and don't affect blood sugar levels as much. Better blood sugar control can be encouraged through picking foods with a lower GL. The glycemic load (GL) accounts for both the food's portion size and glycemic index. It gives a more precise indication of how a food actually affects blood sugar levels. In general, lower GL foods tend to be preferred because they have less of an impact on blood sugar.

Fiber And Blood Sugar Control:

A type of carbohydrate called fiber is one that the body is unable to completely digest. It promotes better blood sugar regulation among other health advantages. Dietary fiber comes in two varieties: soluble fiber and insoluble fiber.

a. Soluble Fiber: In the gastrointestinal tract, soluble fiber develops into a gel-like substance after dissolving in water.

This type of fiber helps slow down digestion, leading to a gradual release of glucose into the bloodstream. Good sources of soluble fiber include oats, barley, legumes, fruits (such as apples and berries), and vegetables (such as Brussels sprouts and carrots).

b. Insoluble Fiber: Insoluble fiber does not dissolve in water and adds bulk to the stool, aiding in digestion and promoting regular bowel movements. While it doesn't directly impact blood sugar levels, it plays a crucial role in overall digestive health. Insoluble fiber can be found in whole grains, nuts, seeds, and many ve getables.

Including a variety of high-fiber foods in your diet can help regulate blood sugar levels, promote satiety, and support overall health.

Portion Control and Timing:

While choosing the right types of carbohydrates is important, portion control and timing also play a role in blood sugar management. Be mindful of the quantity of carbohydrates consumed at each meal and snack. Distribute carbohydrates evenly throughout the day to prevent large spikes or drops in blood sugar levels.

Individualized Approaches:

It's important to note that everyone's response to carbohydrates may vary. Factors such as age, activity level, medications, and individual metabolism can influence how the body processes carbohydrates. Some individuals may benefit from more structured carbohydrate counting or meal planning approaches, which can be tailored to their specific needs and preferences. Consulting with a registered dietitian can provide personalized guidance in managing carbohydrate intake for optimal blood sugar control.

Importance Of Fiber:

Fiber is an indigestible carbohydrate found in plant-based foods, such as fruits, vegetables, whole grains, legumes, nuts, and seeds. Despite being indigestible, fiber offers numerous health benefits:

a. Promotes Digestive Health: Fiber adds bulk to the stool and aids in maintaining regular bowel movements. It can help prevent constipation and promote a healthy digestive system.

b. Blood Sugar Control: Soluble fiber slows down the absorption of glucose, preventing rapid spikes in blood sugar levels after meals. This can be particularly beneficial for individuals with prediabetes or diabetes.

c. Weight Management: High-fiber foods tend to be more filling, which can help control appetite and support weight management efforts. Fiber-rich foods take longer to chew and digest, contributing to a feeling of fullness and satisfaction.

d. Heart Health: Certain types of fiber, such as soluble fiber, have been shown to help lower cholesterol levels, reducing the risk of heart disease.

e. Gut Health: Fiber acts as a prebiotic, nourishing the beneficial bacteria in the gut. A healthy gut micro biome is associated with improved immune function and overall well-being.

To increase fiber intake, focus on incorporating a variety of fiber-rich foods into your diet. Aim for at least 25-30 grams of fiber per day from whole foods, rather than relying on fiber supplements.

Healthy Fats And Protein:

Including healthy fats and adequate protein in your diet is crucial for overall health and well-being:

a. Healthy Fats: Healthy fats, such as monounsaturated and polyunsaturated fats, are essential for various bodily functions and provide numerous health benefits. They support brain health, hormone production, and nutrient absorption. Sources of healthy fats include avocados, nuts, seeds, olive oil, fatty fish (like salmon and sardines), and plant-based oils. It is important to consume these fats in moderation, as they are calorie-dense.

b. Protein: Protein is an essential macronutrient that plays a vital role in building and repairing tissues, supporting immune function, and producing enzymes and hormones. Including adequate protein in your diet can help promote satiety, support muscle health, and aid in weight management. Good sources of protein include lean meats, poultry, fish, eggs, dairy products, legumes, and plant-based sources such as tofu and tempeh.

Balancing your meals with healthy fats and protein helps provide sustained energy, promote satiety, and support overall health and well-being.

Portion Control And Mindful Eating:

Portion control and mindful eating are essential practices for maintaining a healthy diet and achieving a balanced lifestyle:

a. Portion Control: Monitoring portion sizes is crucial to ensure you are not overeating or consuming excessive calories. Be mindful of recommended serving sizes, use measuring tools when necessary, and be aware of your own hunger and fullness cues. Portion control is particularly important when it comes to calorie-dense foods and beverages, such as fats, oils, sweets, and sugary drinks.

a. Mindful Eating: Mindful eating entails being fully present when eating and paying close attention to the process. Take your time, enjoy every bite, and pay attention to the flavor, crunch, and aroma of your food. Eat until you are satiated but not overstuffed by paying attention to your body's hunger and fullness cues. You can have a better relationship with food, eat less excessively, and make more thoughtful decisions by engaging in mindful eating.

MEAL PLANNING AND PREPPING

Creating A Meal Plan:

A meal plan serves as a roadmap for your week ahead, ensuring that you have nutritious and well-balanced meals ready. Here's how to create an effective meal plan:

a. Assess Your Needs: Consider your dietary goals, nutritional requirements, and any specific dietary restrictions or preferences. Determine the number of meals you need to plan for each day and the portion sizes.

b. Variety and Balance: Aim for variety by including a mix of lean proteins, whole grains, fruits, vegetables, and healthy fats in your meal plan. Strive for balance by ensuring that each meal contains a good balance of macronutrients (carbohydrates, protein, and fats).

c. Plan for Success: Consider your schedule, cooking abilities, and available time. Plan meals that are practical and achievable based on your lifestyle. Look for recipes that are quick, simple, and can be prepared in advance.

Grocery Shopping Tips:

Effective grocery shopping plays a crucial role in maintaining a well-stocked kitchen and following your meal plan. Consider these tips to make your grocery shopping experience successful:

a. Make a List: Before heading to the grocery store, create a detailed list based on your meal plan. This helps you stay focused and avoid impulsive purchases.

b. Shop the Perimeter: The perimeter of the grocery store typically contains fresh produce, meats, dairy products, and whole foods. Focus on these areas to ensure a nutrient-dense and wholesome selection.

c. Read Labels: When purchasing packaged foods, read the labels to check for added sugars, unhealthy fats, and artificial additives. Choose products with minimal ingredients and opt for whole food alternatives when possible.

d. Shop Seasonally: Seasonal produce tends to be fresher, more flavorful, and often more affordable. Incorporating seasonal fruits and vegetables can add variety and save money.

Meal Prepping Strategies:

Meal prepping involves preparing meals or meal components in advance to save time during the week. Here are some strategies for effective meal prepping:

a. Plan Your Prep Day: Dedicate a specific day or time each week for meal prepping. This allows you to focus on batch cooking, chopping vegetables, cooking grains, and assembling meal components.

b. Cook in Bulk: Prepare larger quantities of staple foods like whole grains, lean proteins, and roasted vegetables. This provides a foundation for creating multiple meals throughout the week.

c. Pre-cut and Store: Wash, chop, and portion out fruits and vegetables to have them readily available for snacks or quick meal additions. Store them in airtight containers or resealable bags in the refrigerator.

d. Pre-portion Meals: Divide cooked meals into individual portions for grab-and-go lunches or dinners. Use meal prep containers or reusable containers to ensure portion control and convenience.

Batch Cooking And Freezing:

Batch cooking involves preparing large quantities of meals or components to freeze and enjoy at a later time. This method can save time and ensure a variety of meals:

a. Choose Freezer-Friendly Recipes: Look for recipes that freeze well and maintain their quality and taste after thawing. Soups, stews, casseroles, and sauces often freeze successfully.

b. Portion and Label: Divide batch-cooked meals into individual or family-sized portions and label them with the name and date. This helps you keep track of what's in the freezer and ensures freshness.

c. Proper Storage: Use freezer-safe containers or bags to store your batch-cooked meals. Remove excess air from bags to prevent freezer burn. Stack containers neatly to maximize space.

d. Thawing and Reheating: Thaw frozen meals in the refrigerator overnight or use the defrost function on your microwave. Reheat meals thoroughly to ensure they reach a safe temperature.

Smart Snacking Options:

Snacking can be a part of a healthy diet when approached mindfully. Consider these smart snacking options:

a. Whole Foods: Opt for nutrient-dense snacks like fresh fruits, vegetables with hummus, yogurt, nuts, seeds, or homemade energy bars. These choices provide essential nutrients and satisfy hunger.

c. Balanced Snacks: Pair carbohydrates with protein or healthy fats for balanced snacking. For example, enjoy apple slices with nut butter or Greek yogurt with berries.

d. Plan Ahead: Include planned snacks in your meal plan to ensure you have nutritious options readily available. Prep snack-sized portions in advance to grab when hunger strikes.

BREAKFAST AND BRUNCH RECIPES

Energizing Breakfast Bowls

Tropical Acai Bowl:

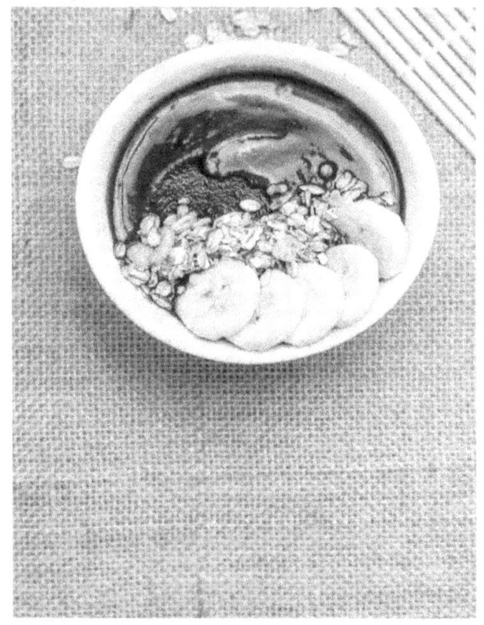

Cook Time: 5 minutes

Servings: 1

Prep Time: 10 minutes

Duration: 15 minutes

Ingredients:

1 frozen acai packet

1 frozen banana

1/2 cup frozen mango chunks

1/2 cup coconut water or almond milk

Toppings: sliced fresh fruits, granola, shredded coconut, chia seeds

Instructions:

Blend the acai packet, frozen banana, frozen mango chunks, and coconut water/almond milk until smooth.

Pour the mixture into a bowl.

Top with your choice of sliced fresh fruits, granola, shredded coconut, and chia seeds.

Berry Quinoa Breakfast Bowl:

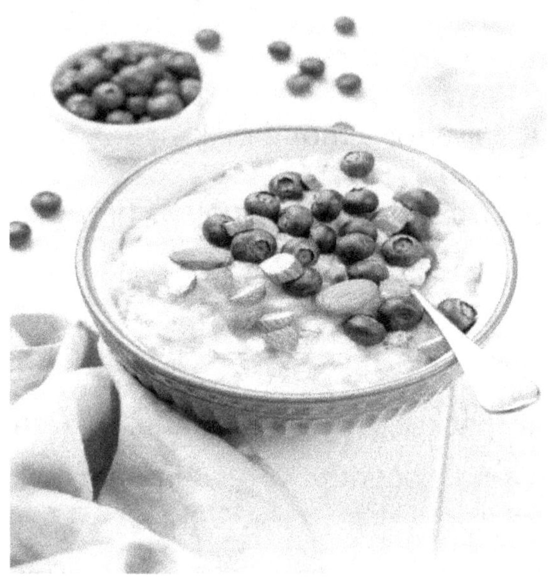

Cook Time: 20 minutes

Servings: 2

Prep Time: 10 minutes

Duration: 30 minutes

Ingredients:

1 cup cooked quinoa

1 cup mixed berries (strawberries, blueberries, raspberries)

1 tablespoon honey or maple syrup

1/4 cup almond milk or Greek yogurt

Toppings: sliced almonds, hemp seeds, mint leaves

Instructions:

In a bowl, mix the cooked quinoa, mixed berries, honey/maple syrup, and almond milk/Greek yogurt.

Divide the mixture into serving bowls.

Garnish with sliced almonds, hemp seeds, and mint leaves.

Green Smoothie Bowl:

Cook Time: 5 minutes

Servings: 1

Prep Time: 5 minutes

Duration: 10 minutes

Ingredients:

1 frozen banana

1 cup spinach

1/2 cup almond milk

1 tablespoon nut butter (almond, peanut, or cashew)

Toppings: sliced banana, granola, chia seeds, coconut flakes

Instructions:

Blend the frozen banana, spinach, almond milk, and nut butter until creamy.

Pour the smoothie into a bowl.

Top with sliced banana, granola, chia seeds, and coconut flakes.

Overnight Chia Pudding Bowl:

Cook Time: 0 minutes

Servings: 1

Prep Time: 5 minutes

Duration: Overnight

Ingredients:

2 tablespoons chia seeds

1/2 cup almond milk or coconut milk

1 tablespoon honey or maple syrup

Toppings: sliced fruits, nuts, seeds, dried coconut

Instructions:

In a jar or bowl, mix the chia seeds, almond milk/coconut milk, and honey/maple syrup.

Stir well and let it sit in the refrigerator overnight.

In the morning, transfer the chia pudding to a bowl.

Top with sliced fruits, nuts, seeds, and dried coconut.

Greek Yogurt Breakfast Bowl:

Cook Time: 0 minutes

Servings: 1

Prep Time: 5 minutes

Duration: 5 minute

1 cup Greek yogurt

1/2 cup mixed berries

1 tablespoon honey or maple syrup

Toppings: granola, sliced almonds, pumpkin seeds

Instructions:

In a bowl, spoon the Greek yogurt.

Top with mixed berries, honey/maple syrup, granola, sliced almonds, and pumpkin seeds.

Peanut Butter Banana Oatmeal Bowl:

Cook Time: 10 minutes

Servings: 1

Prep Time: 5 minutes

Duration: 15 minutes

Ingredients:

1/2 cup rolled oats

1 cup water or milk (dairy or plant-based)

1 tablespoon peanut butter

1 banana, sliced

Toppings: chopped nuts, drizzle of honey, cinnamon

Instructions:

Cook the rolled oats with water or milk according to the package instructions.

Once cooked, stir in the peanut butter until well combined.

Transfer the oatmeal to a bowl.

Top with sliced banana, chopped nuts, a drizzle of honey, and a sprinkle of cinnamon.

Mexican Breakfast Bowl:

Cook Time: 15 minutes

Servings: 2

Prep Time: 10 minutes

Duration: 25 minutes

Ingredients:

1 cup cooked quinoa or brown rice

1 avocado, sliced

1 cup black beans, rinsed and drained

Salsa or pico de gallo

Toppings: cilantro, lime wedges, sliced jalapenos, Greek yogurt (optional)

Instructions:

In a bowl, layer the cooked quinoa or brown rice, avocado slices, and black beans.

Top with salsa or pico de gallo.

Garnish with cilantro, lime wedges, sliced jalapenos, and a dollop of Greek yogurt if desired.

Mediterranean Egg Breakfast Bowl:

Cook Time: 15 minutes

Servings: 1

Prep Time: 10 minutes

Duration: 25 minutes

Ingredients:

2 eggs, boiled or poached

1 cup mixed salad greens

1/4 cup cherry tomatoes, halved

1/4 cup cucumber, diced

Kalamata olives, pitted and sliced

Feta cheese, crumbled

42

Toppings: extra virgin olive oil, lemon juice, dried oregano

Instructions:

Arrange the mixed salad greens in a bowl.

Add the boiled or poached eggs, cherry tomatoes, cucumber, Kalamata olives, and crumbled feta cheese.

Drizzle with extra virgin olive oil, lemon juice, and a sprinkle of dried oregano.

enjoy

Flavorful Omelets And Frittatas

Spinach and Feta Omelet:

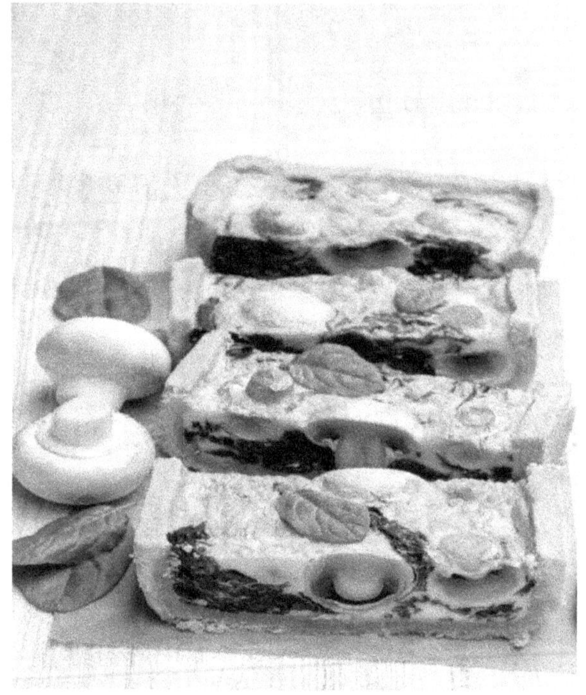

Cook Time: 10 minutes

Servings: 1

Prep Time: 5 minutes

Duration: 15 minutes

Ingredients:

3 large eggs

1 cup fresh spinach, chopped

1/4 cup crumbled feta cheese

pepper and salt as desired

1/9 cup olive oil

Instructions:

In a bowl, beat the eggs thoroughly. Add salt and pepper to taste.

In a nonstick skillet over medium heat, warm the olive oil.

To the skillet, add the spinach, cut it, and cook until wilted for one minute.

In order to spread the eggs equitably, pour the beaten eggs into the skillet and swirl the pan.

The omelet should be cooked for a few minutes until it is set but the top is still a little runny.

Over one half of the omelet, scatter the feta cheese crumbles.

Overlap the extra piece with the cheese.

Cook for a further minute to enable the cheese to melt.

Slide the omelet onto a plate and serve.

Mushroom and Swiss Cheese Frittata:

Cook Time: 20 minutes

Servings: 4

Prep Time: 10 minutes

Duration: 30 minutes

Ingredients:

8 large eggs

1 cup sliced mushrooms

1/2 cup shredded Swiss cheese

14 cup finely minced fresh parsley

Add salt and pepper as desired.

Olive oil, 1 tbsp

Instructions:

Set the oven's temperature to 350°F (175°C).

To thoroughly beat the eggs, whisk them in a big bowl. Add salt and pepper to taste.

In an oven-safe skillet set over medium heat, warm the olive oil.

Sliced mushrooms should be added to the skillet and cooked in order to release moisture and become soft.

The beaten eggs should be added to the skillet and distributed over the mushrooms in a uniform layer.

Over the eggs, strew Swiss cheese crumbles and parsley sprigs.

When the frittata is set in the center, place the pan in the preheated oven and bake for 15-20 minutes.

Remove from the oven, let it cool slightly, then slice and serve.

Mediterranean Vegetable Omelet:

Cook Time: 15 minutes

Servings: 2

Prep Time: 10 minutes

Duration: 25 minutes

Ingredients:

4 large eggs

1/2 cup diced bell peppers (red, yellow, and green)

1/4 cup diced red onion

1/4 cup diced tomatoes

2 tablespoons chopped fresh basil

pepper and salt as desired

Olive oil, 1 tbsp

Instructions:

In a bowl, beat the eggs vigorously. Add salt and pepper to taste.

In a nonstick skillet over medium heat, warm the olive oil.

Add the diced bell peppers and red onion to the skillet. Sauté for a few minutes until slightly softened.

Pour the beaten eggs into the skillet, swirling the pan to distribute them evenly.

Sprinkle the diced tomatoes and chopped fresh basil over one half of the omelet.

Cook for a few minutes until the omelet is set but still slightly runny on top.

Fold the other half over the vegetables.

Cook for another minute until the omelet is fully cooked.

Slide the omelet onto a plate and serve.

Bacon and Cheddar Frittata:

Cook Time: 25 minutes

Servings: 6

Prep Time: 10 minutes

Duration: 35 minutes

Ingredients:

8 large eggs

1/2 cup cooked and crumbled bacon

1/2 cup shredded cheddar cheese

1/4 cup chopped green onions

Salt and pepper to taste

1 tablespoon butter

Instructions:

Preheat the oven to 350°F (175°C).

In a large bowl, whisk the eggs until well beaten. Season with salt and pepper.

Stir in the crumbled bacon, shredded cheddar cheese, and chopped green onions.

Melt the butter in an oven-safe skillet over medium heat.

Pour the egg mixture into the skillet, evenly distributing the ingredients.

Cook on the stovetop for a few minutes until the edges start to set.

Transfer the skillet to the preheated oven and bake for 20-25 minutes until the frittata is set in the center.

Remove from the oven, let it cool slightly, then slice and serve.

Tomato and Basil Omelet:

Cook Time: 10 minutes

Servings: 1

Prep Time: 5 minutes

Duration: 15 minutes

Ingredients:

3 large eggs

1/2 cup diced tomatoes

2 tablespoons chopped fresh basil

Salt and pepper to taste

1 teaspoon olive oil

Instructions:

In a bowl, whisk the eggs until well beaten. Season with salt and pepper.

Heat the olive oil in a non-stick skillet over medium heat.

Add the diced tomatoes to the skillet and sauté for a minute until slightly softened.

Pour the beaten eggs into the skillet, swirling the pan to distribute them evenly.

Sprinkle the chopped fresh basil over one half of the omelet.

Cook for a few minutes until the omelet is set but still slightly runny on top.

Fold the other half over the basil.

Cook for another minute until the omelet is fully cooked.

Slide the omelet onto a plate and serve.

NUTRITIOUS SMOOTHIES AND SHAKES:

Green Detox Smoothie:

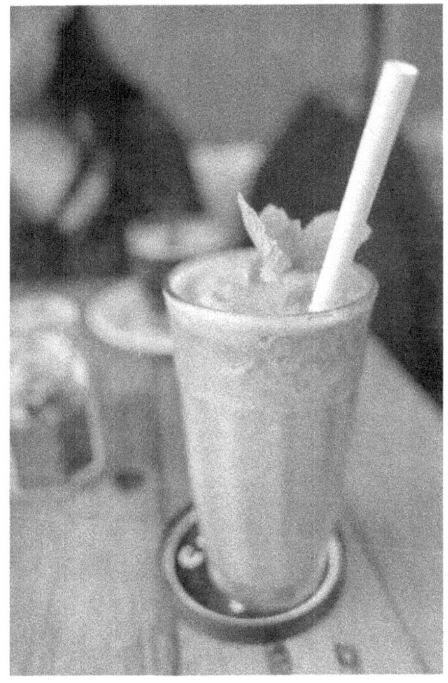

Cook Time: 5 minutes

Servings: 1

Prep Time: 5 minutes

Duration: 10 minutes

Ingredients:

53

1 cup spinach

1/2 cucumber, peeled and chopped

1/2 banana

1/2 cup coconut water or almond milk

1 tablespoon chia seeds

Optional: honey or maple syrup for sweetness

Instructions:

In a blender, combine the spinach, cucumber, banana, coconut water or almond milk, and chia seeds.

Blend until smooth and creamy.

If desired, add honey or maple syrup for sweetness.

Pour into a glass and serve.

Berry Blast Smoothie:

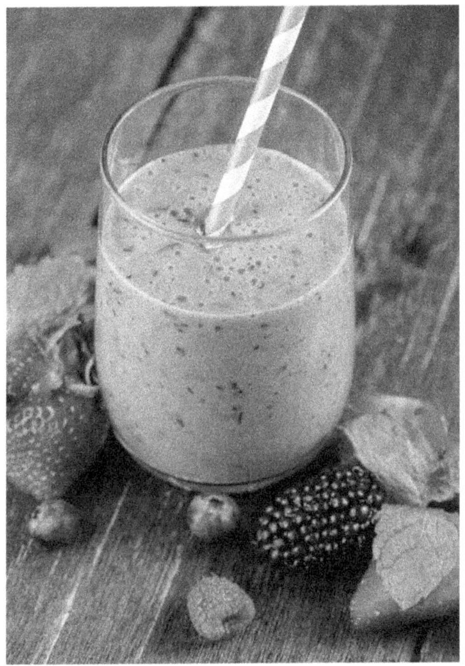

Cook Time: 5 minutes

Servings: 1

Prep Time: 5 minutes

Duration: 10 minutes

Ingredients:

1 cup mixed berries (strawberries, blueberries, raspberries)

1/2 cup Greek yogurt

1/2 cup almond milk or coconut water

1 tablespoon honey or maple syrup

Optional: a handful of spinach or kale

Instructions:

In a blender, combine the mixed berries, Greek yogurt, almond milk or coconut water, and honey or maple syrup.

If desired, add a handful of spinach or kale for added nutrition.

Blend until smooth and creamy.

Pour into a glass and serve.

Tropical Mango Smoothie:

Cook Time: 5 minutes

Servings: 1

Prep Time: 5 minutes

Duration: 10 minutes

Ingredients:

1 ripe mango, peeled and chopped

1/2 cup pineapple chunks

1/2 cup Greek yogurt

1/2 cup coconut water or orange juice

Optional: a squeeze of lime juice and a handful of ice

Instructions:

In a blender, combine the ripe mango, pineapple chunks, Greek yogurt, and coconut water or orange juice.

If desired, add a squeeze of lime juice and a handful of ice for a refreshing taste.

Blend until smooth and creamy.

Pour into a glass and serve.

Peanut Butter Banana Protein Shake:

Cook Time: 5 minutes

Servings: 1

Prep Time: 5 minutes

Duration: 10 minutes

Ingredients:

1 ripe banana

1 cup milk (dairy or plant-based)

2 tablespoons peanut butter

1 tablespoon honey or maple syrup

1 scoop of protein powder (optional)

Optional: a handful of ice

Instructions:

In a blender, combine the ripe banana, milk, peanut butter, honey or maple syrup, and protein powder, if using.

If desired, add a handful of ice for a thicker and colder shake.

Blend until smooth and creamy.

Pour into a glass and serve.

Chocolate Avocado Protein Smoothie:

Cook Time: 5 minutes

Servings: 1

Prep Time: 5 minutes

Duration: 10 minutes

Ingredients:

1/2 avocado

1 cup almond milk or coconut milk

1 tablespoon cocoa powder

1 tablespoon honey or maple syrup

1 scoop of chocolate protein powder

Optional: a handful of spinach or kale

Instructions:

In a blender, combine the avocado, almond milk or coconut milk, cocoa powder, honey or maple syrup, and chocolate protein powder.

If desired, add a handful of spinach or kale for added nutrition.

Blend until smooth and creamy.

Pour into a glass and serve

LUNCH AND DINNER RECIPES

Nourishing Soups And Salads
Urishing Soups:

Lentil Soup:

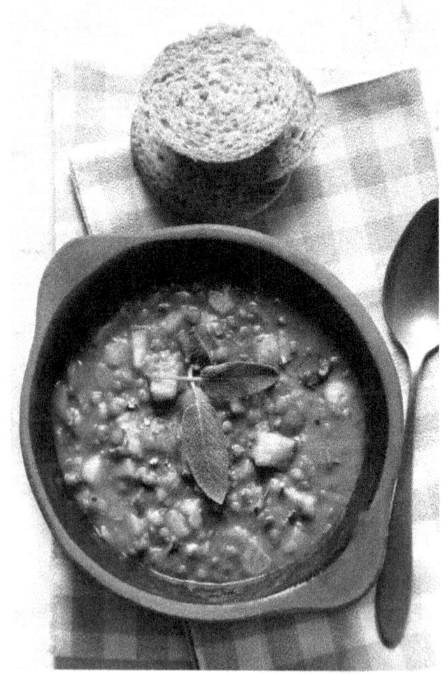

Cook Time: 40 minutes

Servings: 4

Prep Time: 10 minutes

Duration: 50 minutes

Ingredients:

1 cup dried lentils

1 onion, diced

2 carrots, diced

2 celery stalks, diced

3 cloves garlic, minced

4 cups vegetable broth

1 teaspoon ground cumin

1/2 teaspoon ground coriander

Salt and pepper to taste

Fresh parsley for garnish

Instructions:

Rinse the lentils and set aside.

In a large pot, heat some oil over medium heat.

Add the onion, carrots, celery, and garlic. Sauté for 5 minutes until softened.

Add the lentils, vegetable broth, cumin, coriander, salt, and pepper.

Bring the soup to a boil, then reduce heat and simmer for about 30 minutes until the lentils are tender.

Adjust the seasoning if needed.

Serve hot, garnished with fresh parsley.

Chicken Noodle Soup:

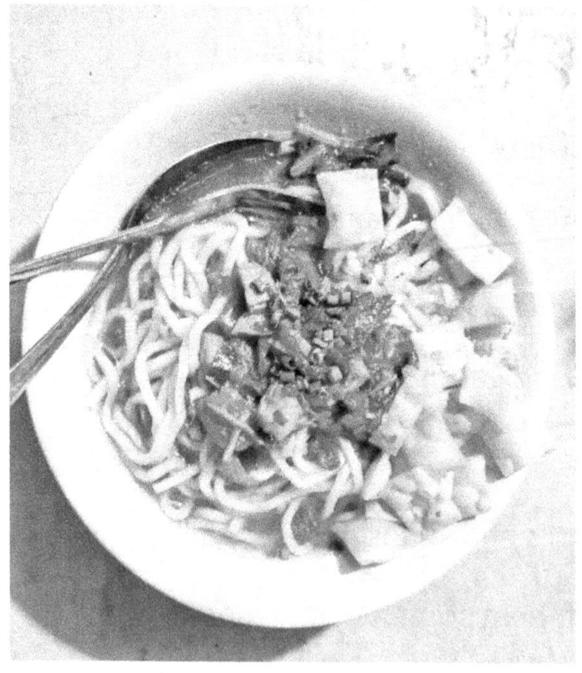

Cook Time: 30 minutes

Servings: 4

Prep Time: 10 minutes

Duration: 40 minutes

Ingredients:

2 chicken breasts, cooked and shredded

6 cups chicken broth

2 carrots, sliced

2 celery stalks, sliced

1 onion, diced

2 cloves garlic, minced

1 cup egg noodles

1 teaspoon dried thyme

Salt and pepper to taste

Fresh parsley for garnish

Instructions:

In a large pot, bring the chicken broth to a boil.

Add the carrots, celery, onion, and garlic. Cook for 5 minutes until vegetables are slightly tender.

Add the shredded chicken, egg noodles, dried thyme, salt, and pepper.

Simmer for about 15-20 minutes until the noodles are cooked and the flavors are well combined.

Adjust the seasoning if needed.

Serve hot, garnished with fresh parsley.

Tomato Basil Soup:

Cook Time: 30 minutes

Servings: 4

Prep Time: 10 minutes

Duration: 40 minutes

Ingredients:

2 cans diced tomatoes

1 onion, diced

3 cloves garlic, minced

4 cups vegetable broth

1/2 cup fresh basil leaves, chopped

1/4 cup heavy cream (optional)

Salt and pepper to taste

Instructions:

In a large pot, sauté the diced onion and minced garlic until softened.

Add the diced tomatoes and vegetable broth to the pot.

Bring the mixture to a boil, then reduce heat and simmer for about 20 minutes.

Using an immersion blender or regular blender, blend the soup until smooth.

Stir in the fresh basil and heavy cream (if using).

Season with salt and pepper to taste.

Heat the soup for another 5 minutes.

Serve hot.

Butternut Squash Soup:

Cook Time: 40 minutes

Servings: 4

Prep Time: 10 minutes

Duratlon: 50 minutes

Ingredients:

1 butternut squash, peeled, seeded, and cubed

1 onion, diced

2 cloves garlic, minced

4 cups vegetable broth

1/2 teaspoon ground cinnamon

1/4 teaspoon ground nutmeg

Salt and pepper to taste

Olive oil for drizzling

Optional toppings: roasted pumpkin seeds, sour cream, fresh herbs

Instructions:

Preheat the oven to 400°F (200°C).

Place the butternut squash cubes on a baking sheet. Drizzle with olive oil and sprinkle with salt and pepper. Toss to coat.

Roast the butternut squash in the preheated oven for 30 minutes until tender and slightly caramelized.

In a large pot, sauté the diced onion and minced garlic until softened.

Add the roasted butternut squash, vegetable broth, ground cinnamon, and ground nutmeg to the pot.

Bring the mixture to a boil, then reduce heat and simmer for about 10 minutes.

Using an immersion blender or regular blender, blend the soup until smooth.

Season with salt and pepper to taste.

Heat the soup for another 5 minutes.

Serve hot, garnished with optional toppings if desired.

Minestrone Soup:

Cook Time: 45 minutes

Servings: 6

Prep Time: 15 minutes

Duration: 60 minutes

Ingredients:

2 tablespoons olive oil

1 onion, diced

3 cloves garlic, minced

2 carrots, diced

2 celery stalks, diced

1 zucchini, diced

1 can diced tomatoes

4 cups vegetable broth

1 can kidney beans, drained and rinsed

1 cup cooked pasta (such as macaroni or shells)

1 teaspoon dried basil

1 teaspoon dried oregano

Salt and pepper to taste

Fresh parsley for garnish

Instructions:

In a large pot, heat the olive oil over medium heat.

Add the diced onion, minced garlic, carrots, celery, and zucchini. Sauté for 5 minutes until the vegetables are slightly softened.

Add the diced tomatoes, vegetable broth, kidney beans, dried basil, dried oregano, salt, and pepper to the pot.

Bring the soup to a boil, then reduce heat and simmer for about 30 minutes until the flavors meld together.

Stir in the cooked pasta.

Adjust the seasoning if needed.

Serve hot, garnished with fresh parsley.

Satisfying Sandwiches and Wraps:

Turkey Avocado Wrap:
Cook Time: 10 minutes

Servings: 2

Prep Time: 10 minutes

Duration: 20 minutes

Ingredients:

4 large tortilla wraps

8 slices of turkey

1 avocado, sliced

1/2 cup baby spinach leaves

2 tablespoons Greek yogurt or mayonnaise

Salt and pepper to taste

Instructions:

Lay out the tortilla wraps on a clean surface.

Spread the Greek yogurt or mayonnaise evenly over the wraps.

Layer each wrap with 2 slices of turkey, avocado slices, and a handful of baby spinach leaves.

Season with salt and pepper to taste.

Roll up the wraps tightly, tucking in the sides as you go.

Cut each wrap in half and serve.

Caprese Panini:

Cook Time: 10 minutes

Servings: 2

Prep Time: 5 minutes

Duration: 15 minutes

Ingredients:

4 slices of ciabatta bread

4 slices of fresh mozzarella cheese

2 tomatoes, sliced

Fresh basil leaves

2 tablespoons balsamic glaze

Salt and pepper to taste

Olive oil for brushing

Instruction

Preheat a panini press or grill pan.

Brush one side of each slice of ciabatta bread with olive oil.

On the other side of the bread, layer a slice of fresh mozzarella cheese, tomato slices, and fresh basil leaves.

Drizzle with balsamic glaze and season with salt and pepper to taste.

Top with another slice of bread, oiled side facing up.

Place the sandwiches in the panini press or grill pan and cook for about 5 minutes until the bread is toasted and the cheese is melted.

Remove from the heat, cut in half, and serve.

Greek Chicken Pita:

Cook Time: 15 minutes

Servings: 2

Prep Time: 10 minutes

Duration: 25 minutes

Ingredients:

2 whole wheat pitas

2 cooked chicken breasts, sliced

1/2 cup diced cucumbers

1/2 cup diced tomatoes

1/4 cup sliced red onions

1/4 cup crumbled feta cheese

2 tablespoons Greek yogurt

1 tablespoon lemon juice

Fresh dill for garnish

Salt and pepper to taste

Instructions:

In a bowl, mix together the Greek yogurt, lemon juice, fresh dill, salt, and pepper.

Open the whole wheat pitas to form pockets.

Spread the Greek yogurt sauce inside each pita pocket.

Fill each pocket with sliced chicken breasts, diced cucumbers, diced tomatoes, sliced red onions, and crumbled feta cheese.

Season with salt and pepper to taste.

Garnish with fresh dill.

Serve.

Vegetarian Quinoa Salad Wrap:
Cook Time: 20 minutes

Servings: 2

Prep Time: 10 minutes

Duration: 30 minutes

Ingredients:

4 large tortilla wraps

1 cup cooked quinoa

1 cup mixed vegetables (such as bell peppers, cucumber, and cherry tomatoes), diced

1/2 cup crumbled feta cheese

2 tablespoons hummus

Fresh herbs (such as parsley or cilantro) for garnish

Salt and pepper to taste

Instructions:

Lay out the tortilla wraps on a clean surface.

Spread 1/2 tablespoon of hummus evenly over each wrap.

In a bowl, mix together the cooked quinoa, diced mixed vegetables, crumbled feta cheese, salt, and pepper.

Spoon the quinoa salad mixture onto each wrap, leaving some space around the edges.

Sprinkle fresh herbs over the filling.

Fold in the sides of the wraps, then roll them up tightly.

Cut each wrap in half and serve.

Wholesome Grain And Vegetable Bowls:

Quinoa and Roasted Vegetable Bowl:

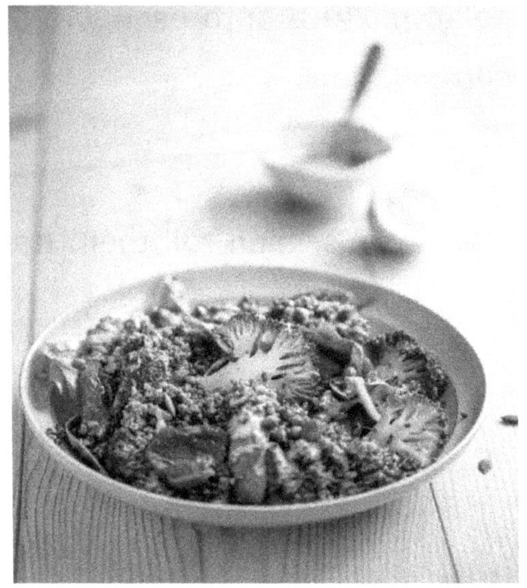

Cook Time: 30 minutes

Servings: 2

Prep Time: 15 minutes

Duration: 45 minutes

Ingredients:

1 cup cooked quinoa

2 cups mixed roasted vegetables (such as bell peppers, zucchini, and sweet potatoes), diced

1 cup baby spinach or kale leaves

1/4 cup crumbled feta cheese

2 tablespoons balsamic vinaigrette

Salt and pepper to taste

Instructions:

In a bowl, combine the cooked quinoa, roasted vegetables, baby spinach or kale leaves, and crumbled feta cheese.

Drizzle with balsamic vinaigrette and toss to coat.

Season with salt and pepper to taste.

Serve warm or at room temperature.

Brown Rice and Teriyaki Tofu Bowl:

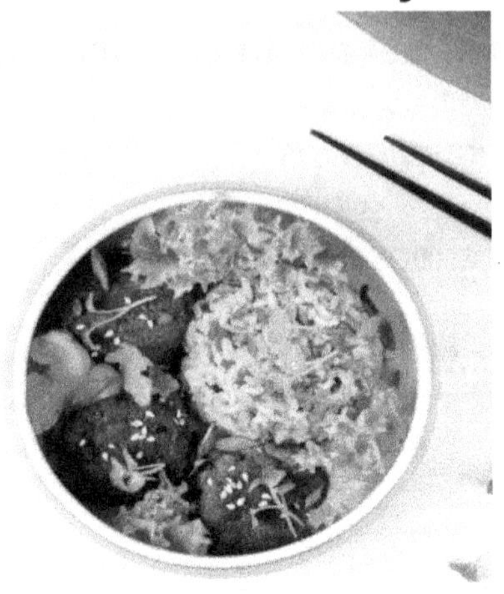

Cook Time: 40 minutes

Servings: 2

Prep Time: 15 minutes

Duration: 55 minutes

Ingredients:

1 cup cooked brown rice

1 cup cubed tofu

2 cups mixed stir-fried vegetables (such as broccoli, bell peppers, and snap peas)

2 tablespoons teriyaki sauce

1 tablespoon sesame seeds

Optional: sliced green onions for garnish

Instructions:

In a non-stick skillet, cook the cubed tofu over medium heat until golden brown.

Add the stir-fried vegetables to the skillet and cook until tender-crisp.

Stir in the teriyaki sauce and cook for an additional minute.

In a bowl, combine the cooked brown rice, tofu, and stir-fried vegetables.

Sprinkle with sesame seeds and garnish with sliced green onions, if desired.

Serve warm.

Quinoa and Chickpea Power Bowl:

Cook Time: 20 minutes

Servings: 2

Prep Time: 10 minutes

Duration: 30 minutes

Ingredients:

1 cup cooked quinoa

1 cup cooked chickpeas

2 cups mixed salad greens

1/2 cucumber, sliced

1/2 cup cherry tomatoes, halved

1/4 cup sliced red onions

2 tablespoons lemon tahini dressing

Salt and pepper to taste

Instructions:

In a bowl, combine the cooked quinoa, cooked chickpeas, mixed salad greens, cucumber slices, cherry tomatoes, and sliced red onions.

Drizzle with lemon tahini dressing and toss to coat.

Season with salt and pepper to taste.

Serve chilled or at room temperature.

Farro and Grilled Vegetable Bowl:

Cook Time: 40 minutes

Servings: 2

Prep Time: 15 minutes

Duration: 55 minutes

Ingredients:

1 cup cooked farro

2 cups mixed grilled vegetables (such as eggplant, zucchini, and asparagus), sliced

1 cup arugula or baby spinach leaves

1/4 cup crumbled goat cheese

2 tablespoons balsamic glaze

Salt and pepper to taste

Instructions:

In a bowl, combine the cooked farro, grilled vegetables, arugula or baby spinach leaves, and crumbled goat cheese.

Drizzle with balsamic glaze and toss to coat.

81

Season with salt and pepper to taste.

Serve warm or at room temperature.

Barley and Roasted Beet Bowl:

Cook Time: 50 minutes

Servings: 2

Prep Time: 15 minutes

Duration: 1 hour 5 minutes

Ingredients:

1 cup cooked barley

2 medium roasted beets, peeled and diced

2 cups mixed salad greens

1/4 cup crumbled feta cheese

2 tablespoons lemon vinaigrette

Salt and pepper to taste

Instructions:

In a bowl, combine the cooked barley, roasted beets, mixed salad greens, and crumbled feta cheese.

Drizzle with lemon vinaigrette and toss to coat.

Season with salt and pepper to taste.

Serve chilled or at room temperature.

Flavorful Poultry and Seafood Dishes:

Lemon Garlic Roasted Chicken:
Cook Time: 1 hour 10 minutes

Servings: 4

Prep Time: 10 minutes

Duration: 1 hour 20 minutes

Ingredients:

4 chicken thighs, bone-in and skin-on

4 cloves garlic, minced

Zest and juice of 1 lemon

2 tablespoons olive oil

1 teaspoon dried thyme

Salt and pepper to taste

Instructions:

83

Preheat the oven to 425°F (220°C).

In a small bowl, combine the minced garlic, lemon zest, lemon juice, olive oil, dried thyme, salt, and pepper.

Place the chicken thighs in a baking dish and pour the lemon garlic mixture over them, making sure they are coated evenly.

Roast in the preheated oven for about 1 hour until the chicken is cooked through and the skin is crispy.

Serve hot.

DELICIOUS VEGETARIAN AND VEGAN OPTIONS

Lentil Curry:

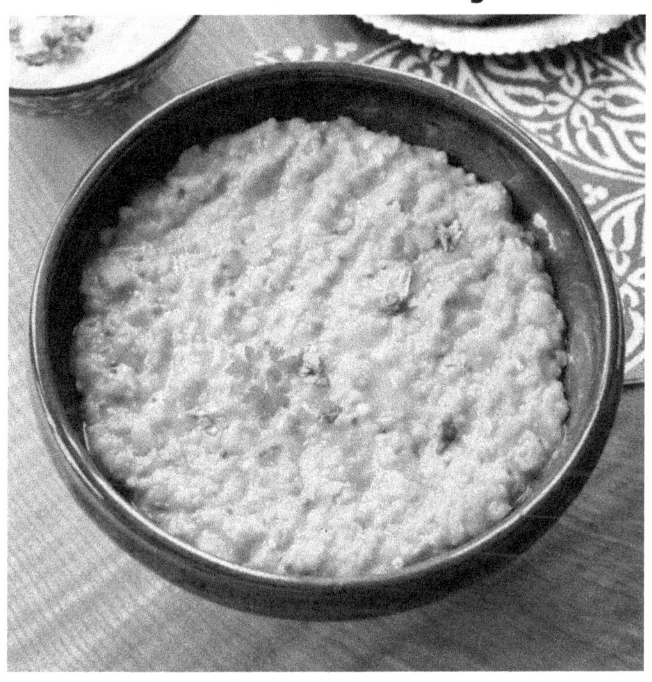

Cook Time: 40 minutes

Servings: 4

Prep Time: 10 minutes

Duration: 50 minutes

Ingredients:

85

1 cup dried lentils

1 onion, diced

3 cloves garlic, minced

1 tablespoon curry powder

1 teaspoon ground cumin

1/2 teaspoon ground turmeric

1 can diced tomatoes

1 can coconut milk

2 cups vegetable broth

Salt and pepper to taste

Fresh cilantro for garnish

Cooked rice or naan bread for serving

Instructions:

Rinse the lentils and set aside.

In a large pot, sauté the diced onion and minced garlic until softened.

Add the curry powder, ground cumin, and ground turmeric. Cook for another minute until fragrant.

Add the lentils, diced tomatoes, coconut milk, vegetable broth, salt, and pepper to the pot.

Bring the mixture to a boil, then reduce heat and simmer for about 30 minutes until the lentils are tender and the flavors meld together.

Adjust the seasoning if needed.

Serve the lentil curry over cooked rice or with naan bread. Garnish with fresh cilantro.

Vegetable Stir-Fry:

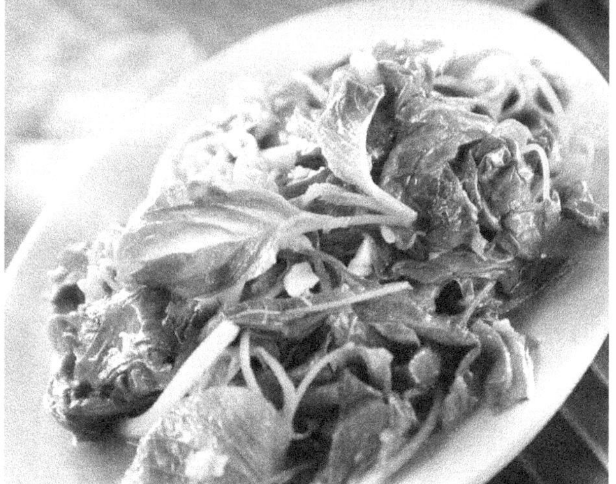

Cook Time: 15 minutes

Servings: 4

Prep Time: 10 minutes

Duration: 25 minutes

Ingredients:

2 tablespoons sesame oil

1 onion, sliced

2 cloves garlic, minced

2 cups mixed vegetables (such as bell peppers, broccoli, and carrots), sliced

1 cup snap peas

1/4 cup soy sauce or tamari

2 tablespoons rice vinegar

1 tablespoon maple syrup or agave nectar

1 tablespoon cornstarch (optional for thickening)

Sesame seeds for garnish

Cooked rice or noodles for serving

Instructions:

Heat the sesame oil in a large skillet or wok over medium-high heat.

Add the sliced onion and minced garlic to the skillet. Cook for about 2-3 minutes until softened.

Add the mixed vegetables and snap peas to the skillet. Stir-fry for another 5-7 minutes until the vegetables are tender-crisp.

In a small bowl, whisk together the soy sauce or tamari, rice vinegar, maple syrup or agave nectar, and cornstarch (if using) until well combined.

Pour the sauce over the vegetables in the skillet and stir to coat evenly. Cook for another minute until the sauce thickens slightly.

Remove from heat and garnish with sesame seeds.

Serve the vegetable stir-fry over cooked rice or noodles.

Chickpea And Vegetable Curry:

Cook Time: 30 minutes

Servings: 4

Prep Time: 10 minutes

Duration: 40 minutes

Ingredients:

1 tablespoon olive oil

1 onion, diced

2 cloves garlic, minced

1 tablespoon curry powder

1 teaspoon ground cumin

1/2 teaspoon ground turmeric

1 can chickpeas, drained and rinsed

2 cups mixed vegetables (such as cauliflower, bell peppers, and peas), chopped

1 can coconut milk

1 cup vegetable broth

Salt and pepper to taste

Fresh cilantro for garnish

Cooked rice or naan bread for serving

Instructions:

Heat the olive oil in a large pot over medium heat.

Add the diced onion and minced garlic to the pot. Sauté for about 5 minutes until softened.

Add the curry powder, ground cumin, and ground turmeric. Cook for another minute until fragrant.

Add the chickpeas, mixed vegetables, coconut milk, vegetable broth, salt, and pepper to the pot.

Bring the mixture to a boil, then reduce heat and simmer for about 20-25 minutes until the vegetables are tender and the flavors meld together.

Adjust the seasoning if needed.

Serve the chickpea and vegetable curry over cooked rice or with naan bread. Garnish with fresh cilantro.

Zucchini Noodles With Pesto:

Cook Time: 10 minutes

Servings: 2

Prep Time: 10 minutes

Duration: 20 minutes

Ingredients:

2 medium zucchinis, spiralized or cut into thin strips

1 cup cherry tomatoes, halved

1/4 cup pine nuts

2 tablespoons nutritional yeast

2 tablespoons olive oil

2 cloves garlic

Juice of 1 lemon

Salt and pepper to taste

Fresh basil leaves for garnish

Instructions:

In a blender or food processor, combine the pine nuts, nutritional yeast, olive oil, garlic, lemon juice, salt, and pepper. Blend until smooth to make the pesto sauce.

In a large skillet, heat some olive oil over medium heat.

Add the zucchini noodles to the skillet and sauté for about 3-4 minutes until they are tender but still have a slight crunch.

Add the cherry tomatoes to the skillet and cook for another minute until they are slightly softened.

Remove the skillet from heat and add the pesto sauce. Toss the noodles and tomatoes until they are coated evenly.

Serve the zucchini noodles with pesto warm, garnished with fresh basil leaves.

Vegan Black Bean Tacos:

Cook Time: 20 minutes

Servings: 4

Prep Time: 10 minutes

Duration: 30 minutes

Ingredients:

1 tablespoon olive oil

1 onion, diced

2 cloves garlic, minced

1 can black beans, drained and rinsed

1 tablespoon chili powder

1 teaspoon ground cumin

1/2 teaspoon smoked paprika

Salt and pepper to taste

8 small corn tortillas

Toppings: sliced avocado, diced tomatoes, shredded lettuce, salsa, vegan sour cream

Instructions:

Heat the olive oil in a skillet over medium heat.

Add the diced onion and minced garlic to the skillet. Sauté for about 5 minutes until softened.

Add the black beans, chili powder, ground cumin, smoked paprika, salt, and pepper to the skillet. Cook for another 5 minutes until the beans are heated through and the flavors meld together.

Warm the corn tortillas in a dry skillet or in the oven.

Fill each tortilla with a spoonful of the black bean mixture.

Top the tacos with sliced avocado, diced tomatoes, shredded lettuce, salsa, and vegan sour cream.

Serve the vegan black bean tacos warm.

SNACKS AND SIDES

Healthy Snack Ideas

Greek Yogurt Parfait:

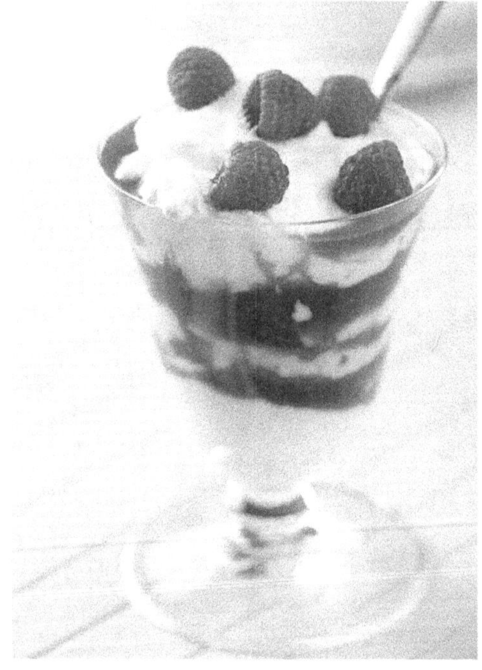

Cook Time: 0 minutes

Servings: 1

Prep Time: 5 minutes

Duration: 5 minutes

Ingredients:

1/2 cup Greek yogurt

1/4 cup fresh berries (such as blueberries or strawberries)

1 tablespoon chopped nuts (such as almonds or walnuts)

1 teaspoon honey or maple syrup (optional)

Instructions:

In a small bowl or glass, layer the Greek yogurt, fresh berries, and chopped nuts.

Drizzle with honey or maple syrup, if desired.

Serve immediately.

Vegetable Sticks with Hummus:

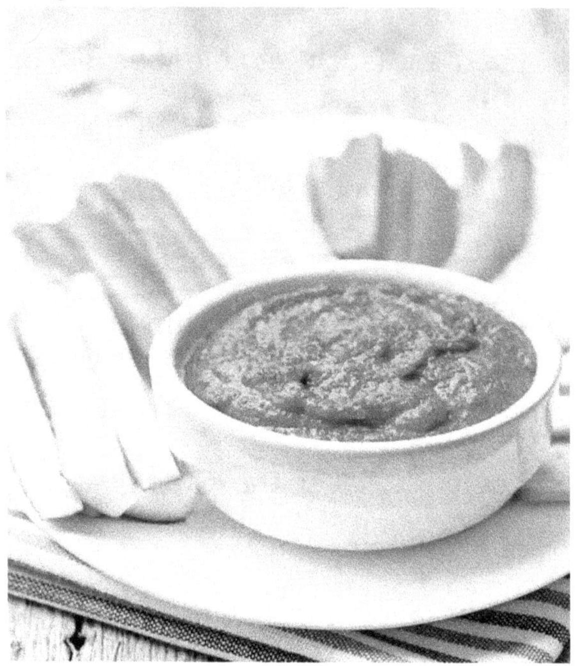

Cook Time: 0 minutes

Servings: 1

Prep Time: 10 minutes

Duration: 10 minutes

Ingredients:

Assorted vegetable sticks (such as carrots, celery, bell peppers, and cucumber)

2 tablespoons hummus

Instructions:

Wash and cut the vegetables into sticks.

Serve the vegetable sticks with hummus for dipping.

Hard-Boiled Egg and Whole Grain Crackers:

Cook Time: 15 minutes

Servings: 1

Prep Time: 5 minutes

Duration: 20 minutes

Ingredients:

1 hard-boiled egg

4-6 whole grain crackers

Instructions:

Cook the hard-boiled egg in boiling water for about 10-12 minutes, then let it cool and peel.

Serve the hard-boiled egg with whole grain crackers.

Apple Slices with Almond Butter:

Cook Time: 0 minutes

Servings: 1

Prep Time: 5 minutes

Duration: 5 minutes

Ingredients:

1 apple, sliced

1 tablespoon almond butter

Instructions:

Wash and slice the apple.

Spread almond butter on the apple slices.

Enjoy!

Avocado Toast:

Cook Time: 5 minutes

Servings: 1

Prep Time: 5 minutes

Duration: 10 minutes

Ingredients:

100

1 slice of whole grain bread

1/2 avocado, mashed

1 teaspoon lemon juice

Salt and pepper to taste

Instructions:

Toast the slice of whole grain bread.

In a small bowl, mash the avocado with lemon juice, salt, and pepper.

Spread the mashed avocado on the toasted bread.

Serve immediately.

Trail Mix:

Cook Time: 0 minutes

Servings: 1

Prep Time: 5 minutes

Duration: 5 minutes

Ingredients:

1/4 cup mixed nuts (such as almonds, cashews, and walnuts)

101

1 tablespoon dried fruit (such as raisins or cranberries)

1 tablespoon dark chocolate chips

Instructions:

In a small bowl, mix together the mixed nuts, dried fruit, and dark chocolate chips.

Enjoy as a healthy snack.

Cottage Cheese with Berries:

Cook Time: 0 minutes

Servings: 1

Prep Time: 5 minutes

Duration: 5 minutes

Ingredients:

1/2 cup cottage cheese

1/4 cup fresh berries (such as strawberries or blueberries)

Instructions:

In a small bowl, combine the cottage cheese and fresh berries.

Serve immediately.

Cucumber and Tomato Salad:

Cook Time: 0 minutes

Servings: 1

Prep Time: 10 minutes

Duration: 10 minutes

Ingredients:

1/2 cucumber, sliced

1/2 cup cherry tomatoes, halved

1 tablespoon olive oil

1 tablespoon balsamic vinegar

Salt and pepper to taste

Instructions:

In a small bowl, combine the cucumber slices and cherry tomato halves.

Drizzle with olive oil and balsamic vinegar.

Season with salt and pepper to taste.

Toss to combine and serve.

103

Edamame:

Cook Time: 5 minutes

Servings: 1

Prep Time: 0 minutes

Duration: 5 minutes

Ingredients:

1/2 cup cooked edamame (in the shell or shelled)

Salt to taste

Instructions:

If using edamame in the shell, cook them in boiling water for about 5 minutes. If using shelled edamame, steam or microwave them according to package instructions.

Sprinkle with salt to taste.

Enjoy as a nutritious snack.

Rice Cakes with Nut Butter:

Cook Time: 0 minutes

Servings: 1

Prep Time: 5 minutes

Duration: 5 minutes

Ingredients:

2 rice cakes

1 tablespoon nut butter (such as almond butter or peanut butter)

1 teaspoon honey or maple syrup (optional)

Instructions:

Spread nut butter on each rice cake.

Drizzle with honey or maple syrup, if desired.

Enjoy!

LIFESTYLE TIPS FOR MANAGING PREDIABETES

Incorporating Physical Activity:

Physical activity is an integral part of managing prediabetes. It helps improve insulin sensitivity, promotes weight loss, and enhances overall cardiovascular health. There are various ways to incorporate physical activity into your daily routine. Here are some examples:

Brisk Walking: Take a 30-minute walk every day. This low-impact exercise is accessible to almost everyone and can be done outdoors or on a treadmill.

Cycling: Ride a bike for 30 minutes a few times a week. Cycling is a great cardiovascular exercise that can be done individually or with friends or family.

Group Exercise Classes: Join group exercise classes such as aerobics, Zumba, or kickboxing. These classes provide structure, motivation, and social interaction.

Strength Training: Incorporate resistance training exercises, such as weightlifting or bodyweight exercises, into your routine. Aim for two to three sessions per week, focusing on different muscle groups.

Swimming: Swim laps or participate in water aerobics classes. Swimming is a low-impact exercise that works the entire body and is suitable for people with joint issues.

Stress Management Techniques:

Stress can negatively impact blood sugar levels and overall well-being. Implementing stress management techniques can help reduce stress and improve diabetes management. Here are some examples:

Deep Breathing: Practice deep breathing exercises by inhaling slowly through your nose, filling your belly with air, and exhaling through your mouth. Deep breathing triggers the relaxation response and helps reduce stress.

Meditation: Set aside a few minutes each day for meditation. Focus on your breath or use guided meditation apps or videos to help calm the mind and relax the body.

Yoga: Engage in yoga practice, which combines physical postures, breathing exercises, and mindfulness. Yoga promotes relaxation, flexibility, and mental well-being.

Hobbies and Relaxing Activities: Engage in activities that bring you joy and help you unwind, such as reading, gardening, listening to music, or practicing a creative hobby like painting or knitting.

Importance Of Sleep And Rest:

Adequate sleep and rest are crucial for overall health and blood sugar management. Here are some practices to prioritize quality sleep:

Stick to a Sleep Schedule: Go to bed and wake up at the same time each day, even on weekends, to regulate your body's internal clock.

Create a Sleep-Friendly Environment: Make your bedroom dark, quiet, and cool. Use blackout curtains, earplugs, or a white noise machine to block external distractions.

Establish a Bedtime Routine: Wind down before bed with a relaxing routine, such as taking a warm bath, reading a book, or practicing relaxation techniques like deep breathing.

Limit Screen Time: Avoid screens, such as smartphones, tablets, and computers, at least an hour before bedtime. The blue light emitted from screens can interfere with sleep.

Monitoring Blood Sugar Levels:

Regular monitoring of blood sugar levels is crucial for managing prediabetes. It allows you to track your progress, identify patterns, and make informed decisions about your lifestyle choices. Here are some monitoring methods:

Self-Monitoring of Blood Glucose (SMBG): Use a glucometer to check your blood sugar levels at home. Your healthcare provider will guide you on when and how often to monitor.

Continuous Glucose Monitoring (CGM): Utilize a wearable device that continuously measures your glucose levels. This provides real-time information and can help you understand the impact of different activities and foods on your blood sugar.

Building A Supportive Network:

Building a supportive network can provide emotional support, accountability, and valuable resources for managing prediabetes. Here are some ways to build a supportive network:

Diabetes Support Groups: Join local or online support groups specifically tailored to individuals with diabetes or prediabetes. These groups provide a platform to connect with others who share similar experiences and challenges.

Healthcare Team: Build a strong relationship with your healthcare team, including your doctor, diabetes educator, and registered dietitian. They can provide guidance, education, and ongoing support.

Family and Friends: Engage family members and close friends in your journey to manage prediabetes. Educate them about your condition and ask for their support in making healthy lifestyle choices.

www.ingramcontent.com/pod-product-compliance
Lightning Source LLC
Chambersburg PA
CBHW050032260726
48658CB00005B/1560